Dr. med. Jakob Derbolowsky

TrophoTraining®
THE WAY I FEEL GOOD

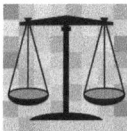

A Quick as a Flash
and Goal-Oriented Relaxation

Foreword

My conversations with people are often about one theme – stress and strong nerves. Many people wish they had less pressure, greater fitness, and more time for the really important things: time for themselves; time for their families, friends and acquaintances; or just time for the beautiful things in life. If this sounds familiar to you, you will surely enjoy this little book – and it will not take you long to read it.

Dr. Jakob Derbolowsky

"If this little book had landed on my desk without your name on it, I would have tossed it aside thinking, it cannot possibly be that simple. Now, I will recommend it to others. I am still amazed that the results were so quick and seemingly effortless."

Professor Dr. Detlev Ploog, former director of the Max Planck Institute of Psychiatry in Munich, Germany

Impressums

Copyright © 2009 by Jakob Derbolowsky
Published in Germany by Psychopädica Verlag, Germering

German Title: TrophoTraining® - So fühle ich mich wohl

Gestaltung und Satz: kggk agentur für gute Kommunikation, Köln
Übersetzung: Emiliy Lemon

Bibliographic information published by the Deutsche Nationalbibliothek

The Deutsche Nationalbibliothek lists this publication in the Deutsche
Nationalbibliografie; Detailed bibliographic data are available in the Internet at
http://dnb.d.nb.de

ISBN 13 978-3-933400-13-0

Dr. med. Jakob Derbolowsky

TrophoTraining®
THE WAY I FEEL GOOD

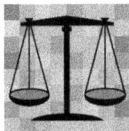

A Quick as a Flash
and Goal-Oriented Relaxation

Contents

Warm up

Dear Readers,

This little book can help you change your life. You can become more independent, open, self-confident, and successful. You will be able to access an unimaginable source of strength and energy that will help you reach all your goals – as long as you really want to ...

Do you feel like a victim of fate or adverse circumstances? Afflicted with illness? Would you like to know what you can do to become the master of your own life? Would you like to find out how you can use an integrated plan to strengthen your physical health, vitality, and emotional balance whenever you want?

You think that it must be extremely difficult and complicated, or even totally impossible? Get ready for a surprise! Everything that you need to do is on these pages. These are small, very simple exercises that can be done easily and quickly wherever you are, with unbelievable and safe results!

You do not have to learn any complicated scientific methodology or study philosophical theories. It is enough if you simply join me for a journey of self-discovery – the duration is only one minute a trip. The best strategy is to start right away – do not wait until you have a quiet moment or you are in the right place. This way, it will soon become part of your daily life and strengthen you. In this book, you will find everything necessary to get started.

TrophoTraining® –
The Secret of Simplicity

So that you do not feel like you have to go into this journey blindfolded, I would like to tell you about a few basic principles that are responsible for the astounding success of this training.

You have probably realized that all of the really big things in our world are very simple in the end. Many great scholars and philosophers came to this conclusion after years of work. In all of the seemingly complicated areas of our lives, it just comes down to exploring the underlying principles deeply enough. Then, from the depths of these principles, you can often achieve an unimaginable amount easily and with little energy.

TrophoTraining® is a scientifically proven method that brings together all of the psychological, psychotherapeutic, and psychoanalytic findings that are **practical** for individuals. It was developed by the author in cooperation with his father, medical doctor and psychoanalyst, Dr. Udo Derbolowsky, who started working with the founder of traditional Autogenic Training, Professor Dr. J.H. Schultz, in 1949. The different *TrophoTraining*® exercises are the result of knowledge and extensive experience gained from decades of medical and scientific work with the human soul, mind, and body. New studies support these results.

Do not be distracted if an exercise seems very easy or even childish or fruitless. The secret to the success of the exercises is, that they are founded on reason, where basic changes cannot be made, and produce something at the heart of human existence, because they address all three dimensions of the individual – body, mind, and soul – in the right manner.

That means that they provide certain images or "mental-emotional messages" through a type of affectionate concentration on certain areas of the body, which then safely and legitimately transforms into physical reality. At no point do you need to "imagine" something that does not exist in reality. You always concentrate on real things, like your body.

Enough theory! Just try it, and you can start looking forward to all the things you will experience through the exercises. Have fun reading and enjoy the first exercise!

The first exercise

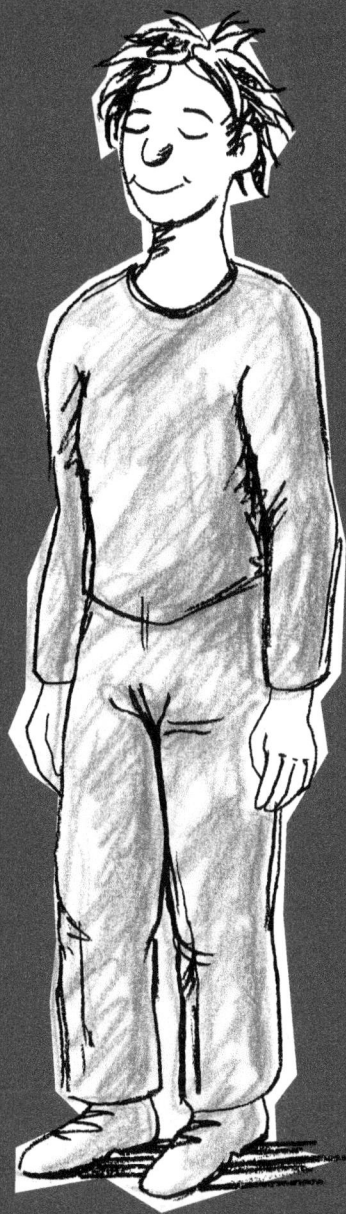

Wherever you are right now, start by paying attention to your breathing. Just pay attention to how the breathing happens entirely on its own. It occurs in three parts: exhalation... pause... inhalation.

And try not to inhale intentionally. Just patiently observe your breathing for three breaths, becoming aware of how it flows into you and out of you again. While you are doing this, imagine how water is poured from a pitcher into a glass. The water flows into the glass from the top, and of course the glass does not fill up from top to bottom, but rather from bottom to top.

Your breathing works the same way. It flows in from above through your nose, but your body fills up from bottom to top, beginning at the buttocks and up to the shoulders.

Let all of your tension flow out with the slowly exhaled breath, as well as everything that emotionally strains you, bothers you, or worries you. Imagine how your slow breathing takes everything

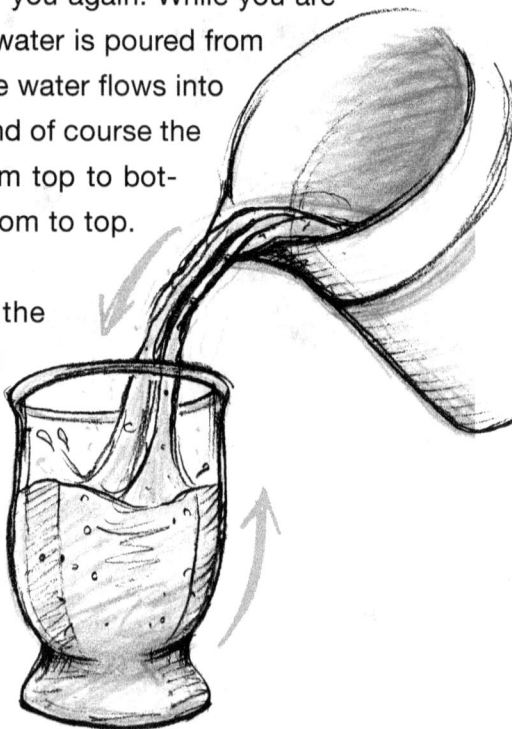

away with it, freeing you of all burdens. I see this process as being similar to draining marshland that is dried out with the help of many trenches. As these channels draw water away, so do your breaths collect your tension and concerns, beginning at the front of the body, flowing around the sides to the back, then running up the neck to the back of the head, over the crown and finally, accompanied by your breath, flowing out of the nose.

Do this exercise for three breaths several times a day for a few days, and as soon as you are concentrating on your breathing, change your thoughts to concentrate on these words:

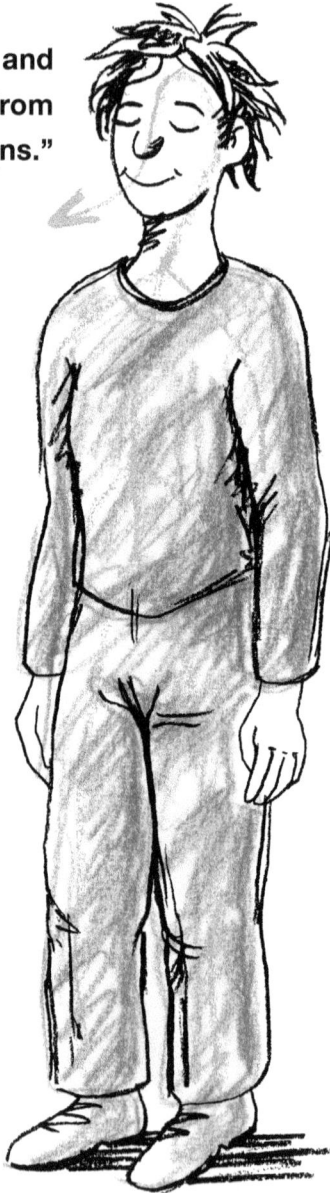

"Refreshed and freed from burdens."

Repeat these words to yourself three times and then finish. You can do it in less than a minute and in any setting, unnoticed by others.

Now close your eyes for a moment and take the time to do this concentration exercise one more time before you continue reading. Repeat this at least three times a day at regular times – before meals, for example – until it becomes a routine for you just like teethbrushing to pause and be aware. Of course you can also do this exercise additionally whenever you are in the mood or if you are experiencing stress.

The second exercise

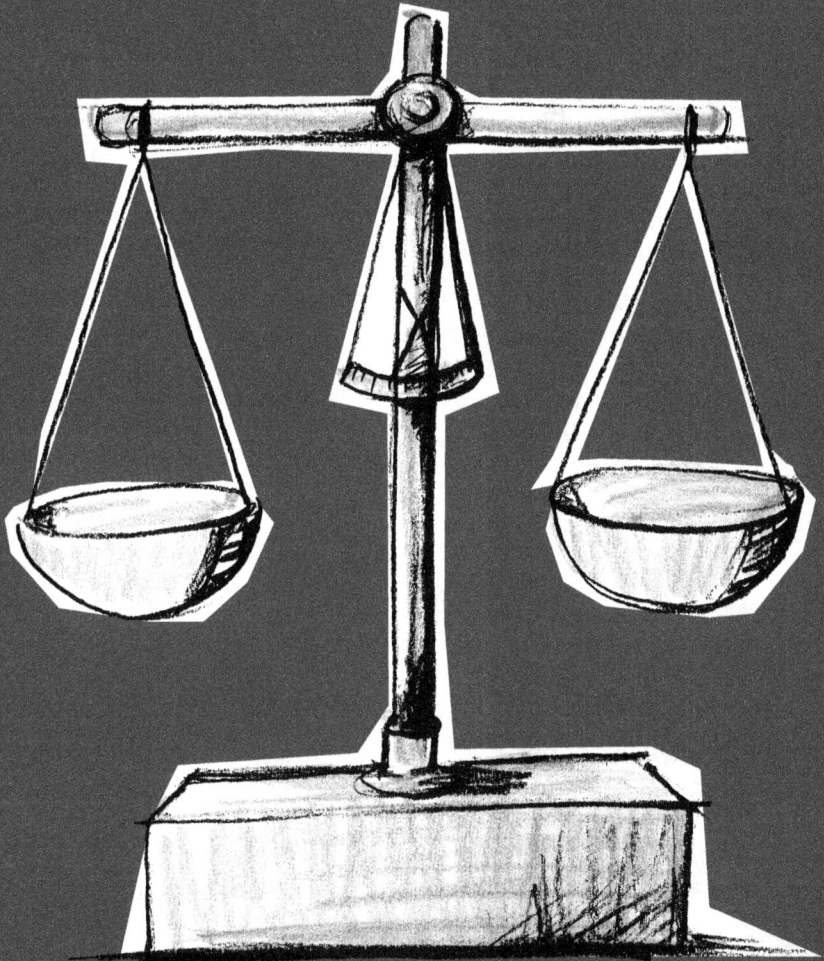

You begin by repeating the first exercise, which you are already familiar with.

Wherever you are, observe your spontaneous breathing. Pack all of your worries, burdens and stresses into the exhaled breath and release them together. Concentrate three times on the words: "Refreshed and freed of burdens." Then add the following sentence and repeat it three times to yourself:

Everything is of equal value.

> (not of **more** value,
>
> not of **less** value,
>
> but of **equal value**).

Connect this sentence to an image: Imagine a scale. A balance scale like those used by pharmacists in the past – two weighing pans, one on the right and one on the left, that are connected by a beam which passes over a fulcrum, and which are in balance when the weight in both pans is equal.

Now imagine that you are on one of the weighing pans everything that is you. On the pan on the other side is everything else, including the demands and annoyances, the stress, even perhaps pain, as well as all the people who want something from you. In other words, everything that is not you and that causes you stress.

Envision both pans hanging at the same level, totally in balance. This is one aspect of reality, that the "inside" and "outside" are equal. Repeat three times to yourself "everything is of equal value." That means "I and everything else" are equal, of equal value, of equal importance. Rejoice in this important realization!

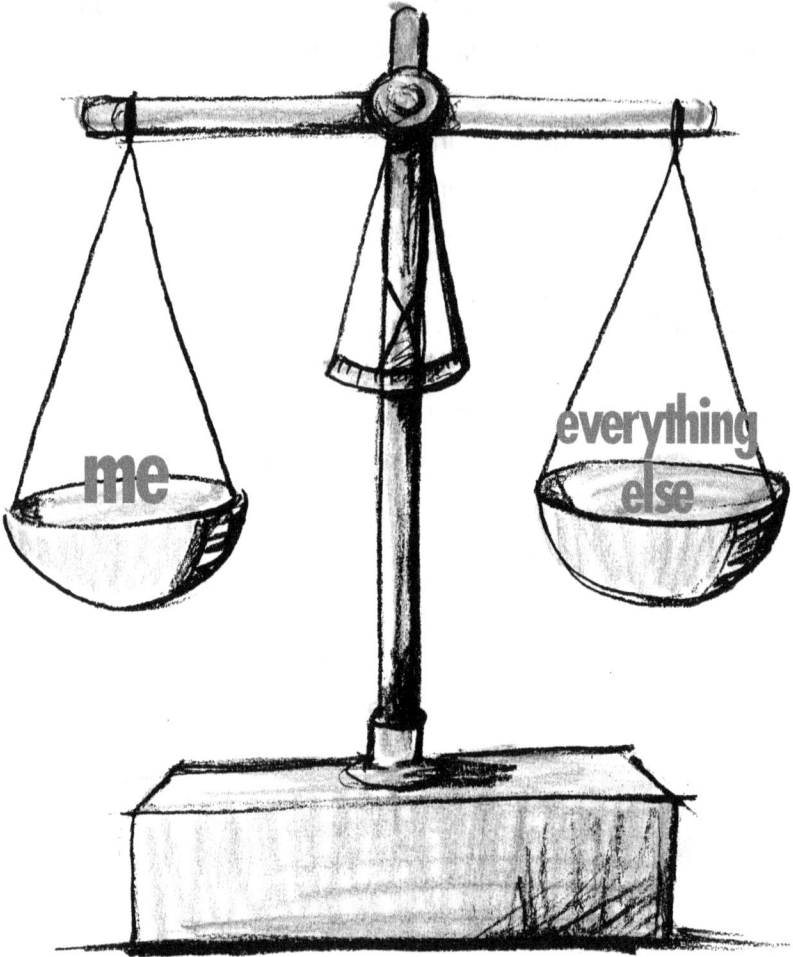

This exercise, like all the other exercises, can be done in any setting, unnoticed by others.

Important: **Please do not do the exercise for longer than a minute, but do it at least three times a day,** for as many days necessary until the image is familiar for you. Then add the next formula and always end your exercises with the thought: "(I am) **refreshed and wide awake."** Very soon, you will see that you can express your opinions and make independent decisions more clearly if you remember this image in day-to-day stressful situations.

The third exercise

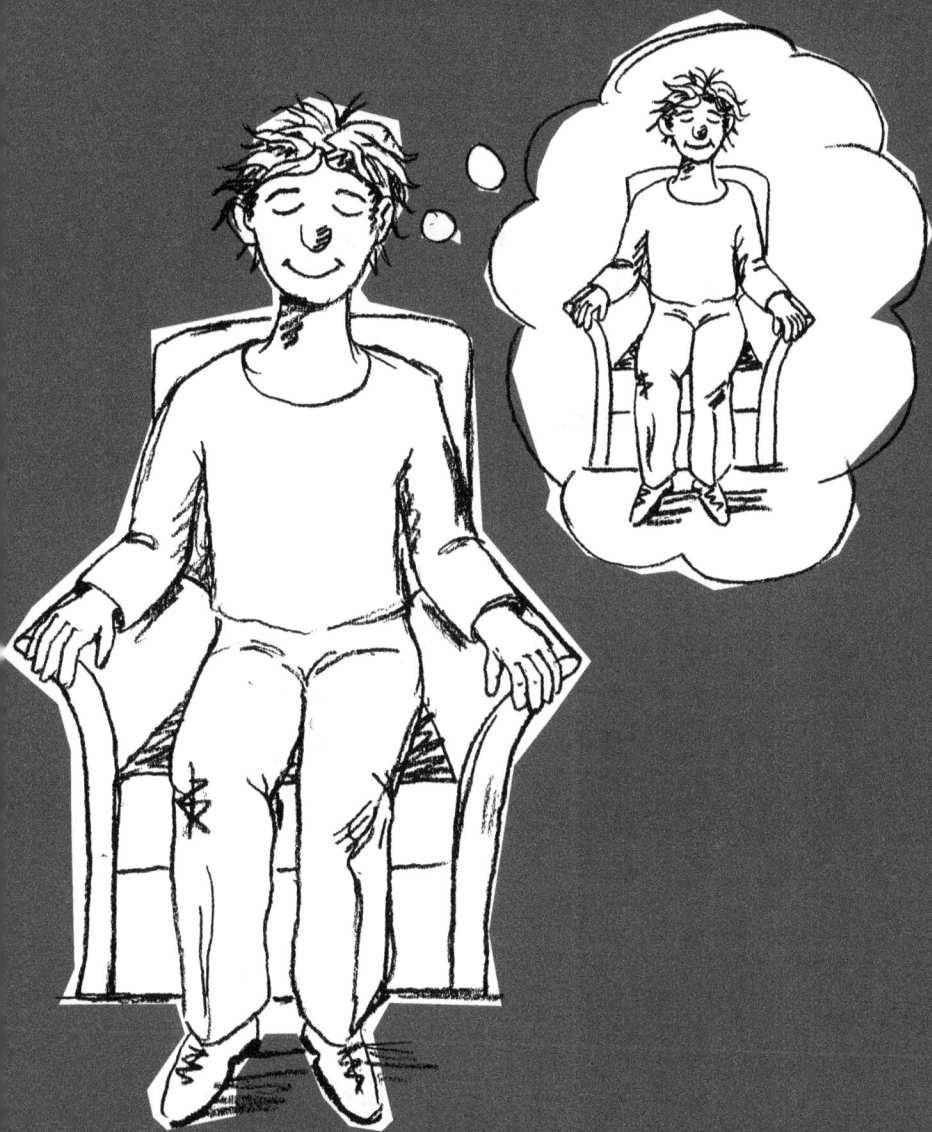

Begin by observing your breathing and again concentrate on the thought, "refreshed and freed of burdens." Imagine again how all the tension, strains, and annoyances flow into your breath and leave your body as you exhale through your nose. Then repeat these words three times in your mind: "... Everything is of equal value ..."

Now be aware of how you – that means your body - are sitting, lying, or standing right now: calm, unmoved. Concentrate on this peaceful image and declare: **"I am really calm, I am really calm, I am really calm"**

After repeating this notion several times you might notice that your subconscious literally conforms to this message, making you calm whenever you think these words. This principle has been proven in numerous scientific investigations.

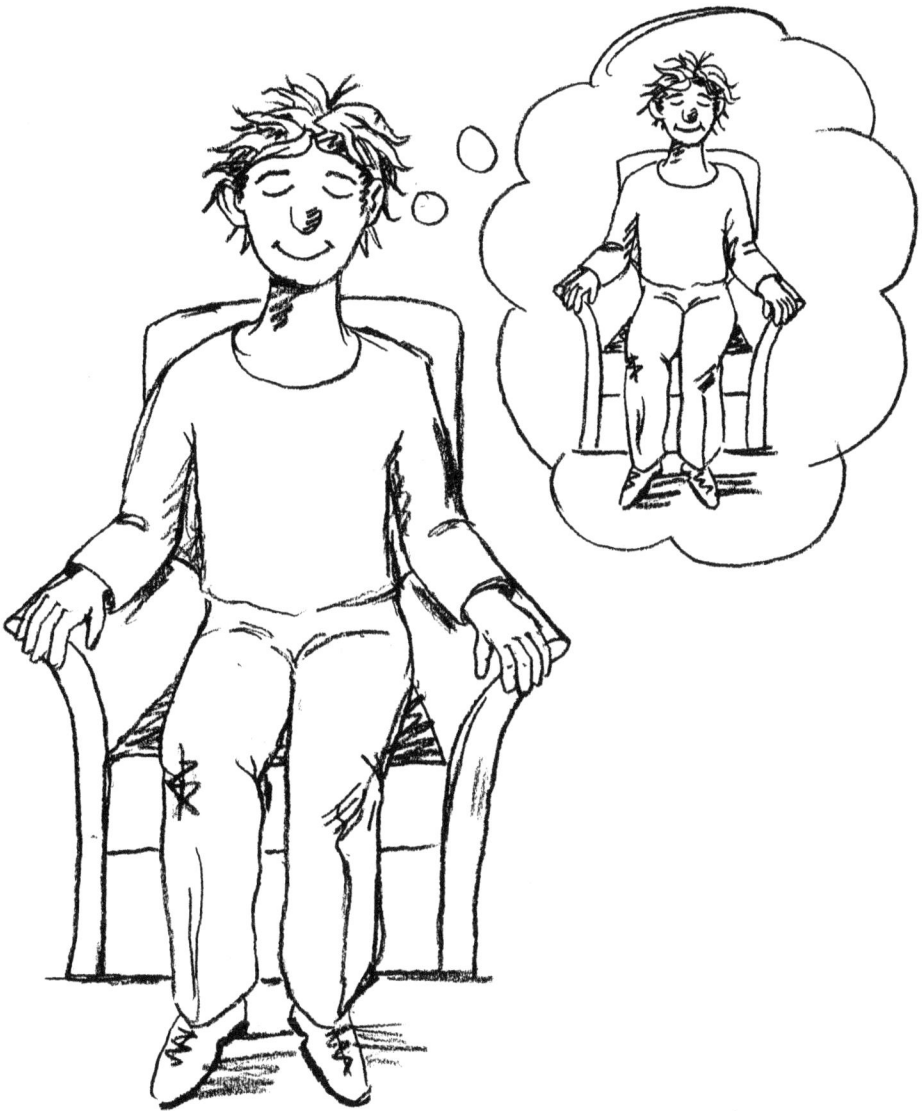

Do this exercise at least three times a day for several days for no longer than about one minute at a time. By repeating this with the previous exercises for a few days before moving on to the next step, you are now well prepared for further exercises in our training.

The fourth exercise

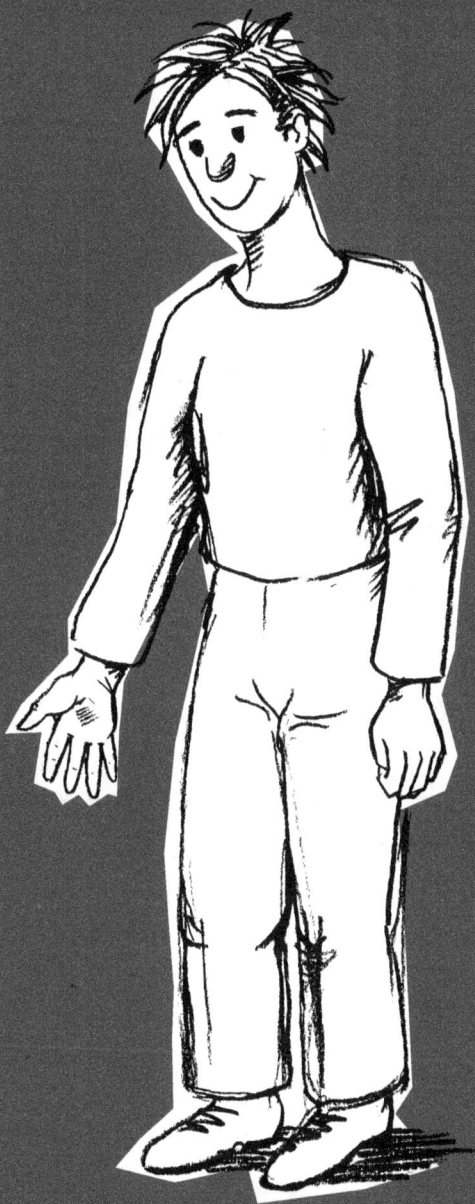

Allow me to ask some unusual questions before we begin with this exercise. What do you think of yourself and your body? Do you like yourself the way you are? Do you ever feel something like gratitude for your body because it has worked so amazingly well for so long, because it is so incredible the way it is?

Why am I asking? I am going to try to answer that without getting lost in the depths of science. You know that the human body usually works well and fulfills all of its tasks without our having to intervene and guide it with our conscious, intelligent and logical mind. So, if this complicated system of cells, organs and regulatory systems – your body – can do its extremely complicated tasks involving the metabolism, energy production, growth, regulation of motion, adjustment to changing circumstances and so much more without requiring our conscious effort, it means that your body must have some kind of intelligence of its own! Many researchers even believe that not only does the entire organism possess a consciousness and intelligence, but so does each individual cell.

And now for the exercise!

Let's apply the concept that the human being is a unit composed of body, mind and soul. There are certain legitimate and measurable relationships between these three "partners" that you have already experienced in your own body and often see in others. For example, think about "when your mouth waters" or about "breaking out in a cold sweat" if something frightening is on your mind, or that "your heart jumps for joy" when imagining something in particular.

These examples are known to be beyond our control because they happen automatically. We experience these reactions; we are at their mercy.

With the findings that *TrophoTraining*® is based on, you can establish inner stability. More than that, you can make a conscious, deliberate, positive impact on your body and mind to strengthen your health, feel better, and experience more joy in life.

Do you want to know how? Well, it is sort of the same as it is with a child. The more attention and love you give the child, the more you do with him and the more lovingly you speak to him, the better your relationship becomes and the closer you will be. So just start speaking to your body in the same way, devote your attention and love to it. In order to become familiar with this technique and practice it, we will start with an area of your body that you know very well – for example, your right arm.

And now you are already at the next exercise phrase:

"My dear right arm, you are heavy and warm."

Please do not think that you have to actively cause something to happen or change something with this phrase. You are simply establishing an objective fact. Because I think you are glad that you have your arm and that your arm weighs several pounds and it is indeed flowing with 98.6 °F blood – even if it feels cool on the outside.

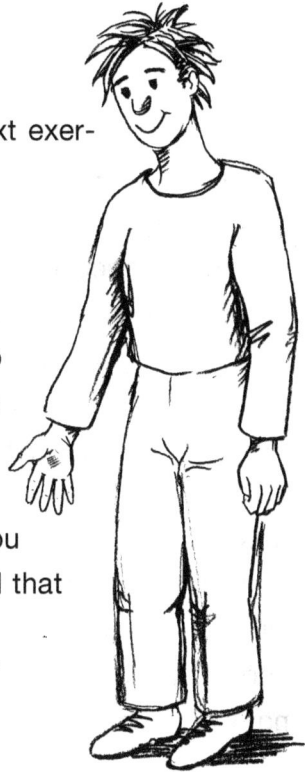

Please resist the temptation to check whether you can feel the weight and warmth of your arm. Usually in Autogenic Training this is taught to be desirable, but in *TrophoTraining*® it is not encouraged. On the contrary, we do not test the result by "feeling" control.

Please keep in mind: The point of this exercise is to establish a more conscious relationship with your body supported by loving thoughts, so later you can also make contact with other specific areas of your organism that may be causing you grief or that you simply want to strengthen.

For now, just imagine that you are communicating something to your arm that you know for certain to be true. The result will only come later. This is similar to sending a letter to a good friend. You know that the reply will come in a few days at the earliest. It is similar with your body. Your body will answer you after you practice the exercise for a while, and then you will clearly feel it. The answer will come; do not worry. Look forward to it!

Finishing the exercise (retraction). When you are finished with your exercise – after about one minute – always return your awareness back to your "external" life by stretching your arms and legs as you do when you wake up in the morning, like a cat stretches after sleep. Then yawn wholeheartedly while saying to yourself: "refreshed and wide awake!" And then open your eyes wide. Do this in the same manner as a cat: stretch and take a deep breath with your mouth, then open your eyes wide and observe your surroundings.

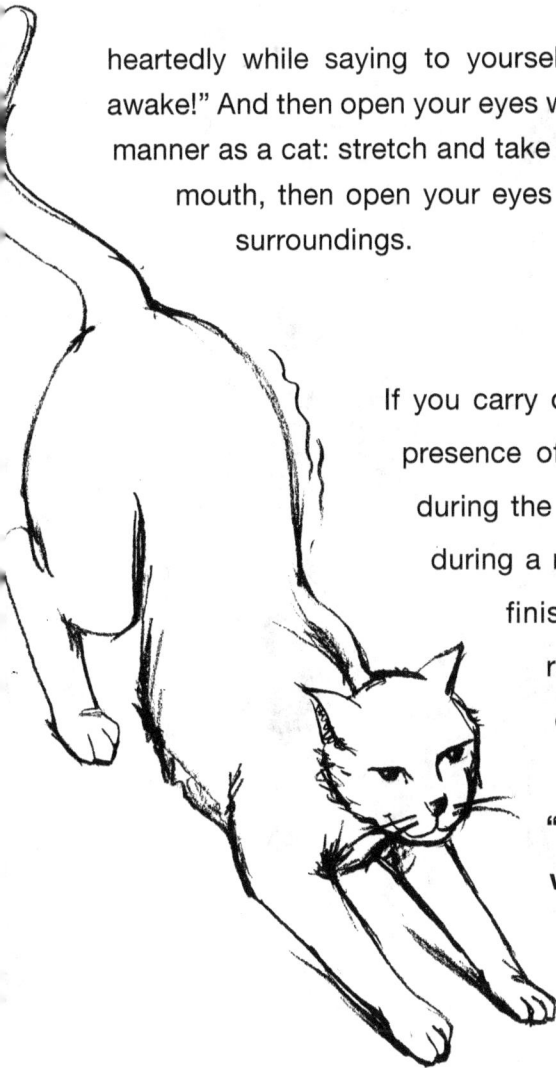

If you carry out the exercises in the presence of others – for example, during the work day, in a concert, during a meeting, or on a train – finish the exercise by repeating silently but energetically to yourself at least three times: **"(I am) refreshed and wide awake!"**

The fifth exercise

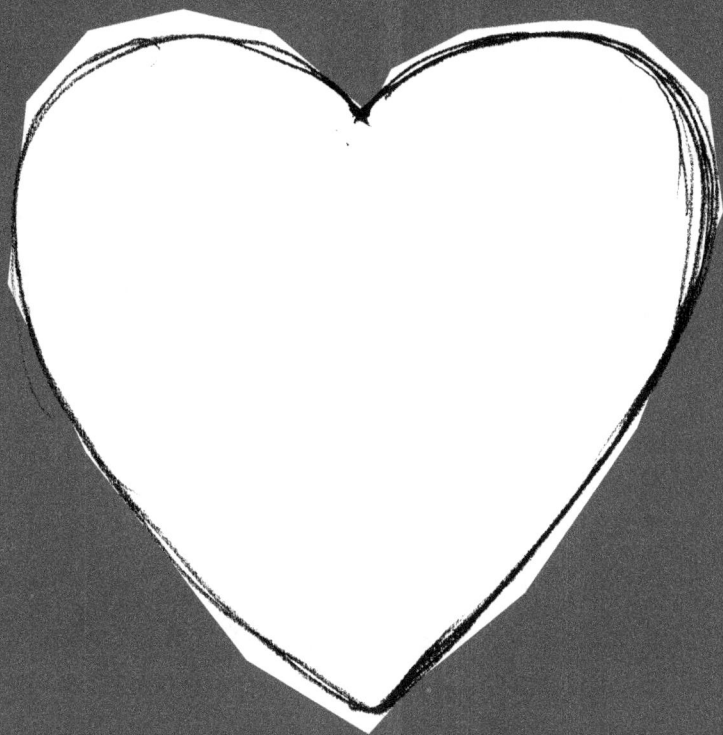

Begin the same way as you are now used to by repeating the earlier phrases:

Everything is of equal value.
I am totally calm.
My dear right arm, you are heavy and warm.

Now send two more messages to your body.
The first one is:

My dear heart, you beat!

I always remind myself how wonderful and calming it is, that this heart – my dear heart – provides my entire body with life-giving nutrients and oxygen day and night and always beats as strongly as is necessary. The important thing is that I embrace this calmly and serenely, because it is indeed doing its work right. And in *TrophoTraining*® a "feeling" proof of the imagination is neither intended nor necessary.

The next phrase is dedicated to breathing:

My dear breath, you come as a gift.

With this message, surrender to the calming knowledge that you do not have to do anything get your breath or to breathe "correctly". Imagine the cloud of oxygen that floods your whole body with every breath. Breathing provides all the cells of your body (about 80 trillion cells!) with new life-energy and removes the waste. The same thing happens for you. Rejoice in it!

The sixth exercise

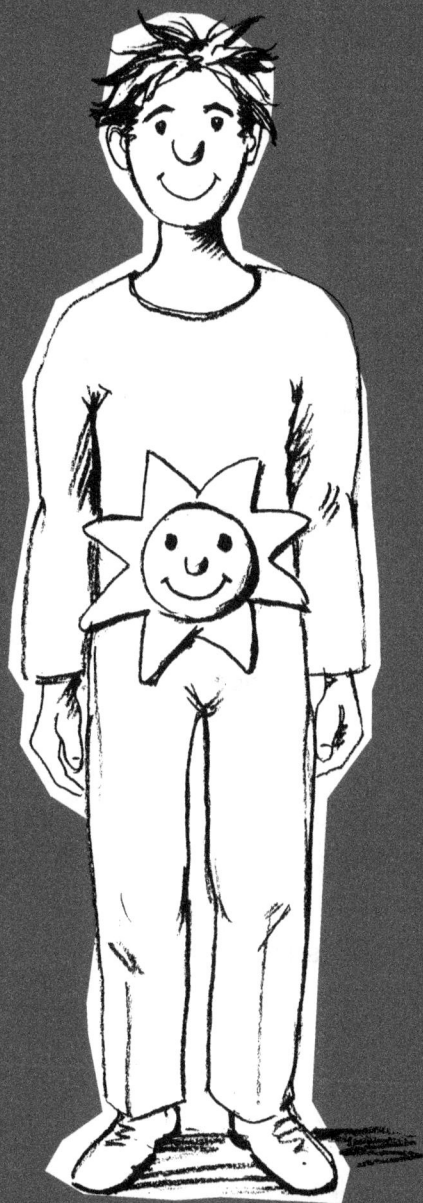

This and the following images are based on the scientific principle that our subconscious does not know logic in the sense of our conscious mind. The subconscious only understands a language of images, sounds and feelings to which it then reacts with unbelievable consistency. Whenever you want to easily achieve or change something with the help of your powerful subconscious, you will be successful if you are able to speak its language. This applies to all of your personal and professional goals, as well as to your body and physical health.

Now back to the exercise. I will suggest several images in the language of the subconscious to deepen communication with your body. As a serious person with a critical mind it may be difficult for you to adopt to this language, because a "language of images and feelings" is inevitably simple, naïve and childish. Of course, you are welcome to think up your own images. To insure the success of these exercises please make sure that the images you select invoke positive feelings in you and that the images are a part of your reality.

I imagine that my body is like a large, well-organized company: At the top is the executive management and below is a management team consisting of "upper, middle, and lower management." Each level of management is responsible for independent decisions and is always the responsible contact point for the others.

Now imagine that your body and its regulatory systems, with the individual organs, glands and cells, are run and managed like a large company. Imagine there is an invisible, energetic management team for every area of your body, every organ, gland, etc., which you can contact in your imagination. In order to address the management personally, give each "organ manager" a name you like and for which you have positive associations.

I have decided to call my organ managers "angels." When I was a child, I felt a close connection to my guardian angel and spoke to him when I needed help. Experience has shown that angel imagery is very effective for most people, because it is readily accepted by the subconscious. And, aside from that, it also creates a connection to the very personal idea of a creator that (almost) everyone has and can trust.

Please give it a try. Your subconscious understands and loves this language. This way you can establish direct and emotional contact with your body and its parts and, when necessary, have a loving effect on it!

Here are the phrases for two more areas of your body. Connect these statements with pleasant emotional images. Practice this along with the previous phrases for several days to become familiar with it.

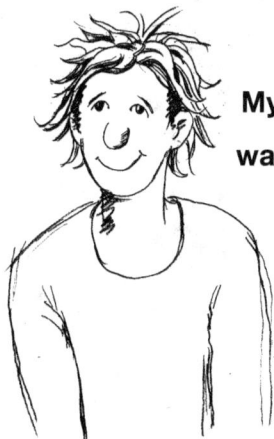

My dear body, you are flowing with warmth.

The body's central heat source is situated in the belly and can be imagined as similar to a warming, springtime sun.

My dear forehead, you are pleasantly cool.

Having a cool head is what we wish for in difficult situations and the coolness is, in fact, present on our forehead where the "heat" exchange takes place. The awareness of a "cool head" is synonymous for being calm.

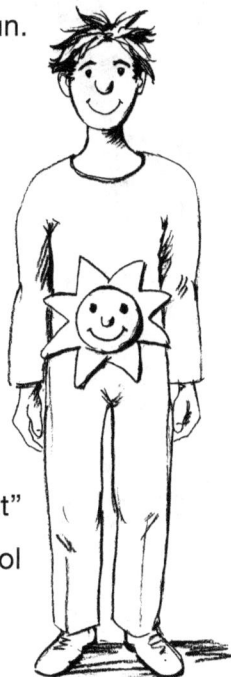

The seventh exercise

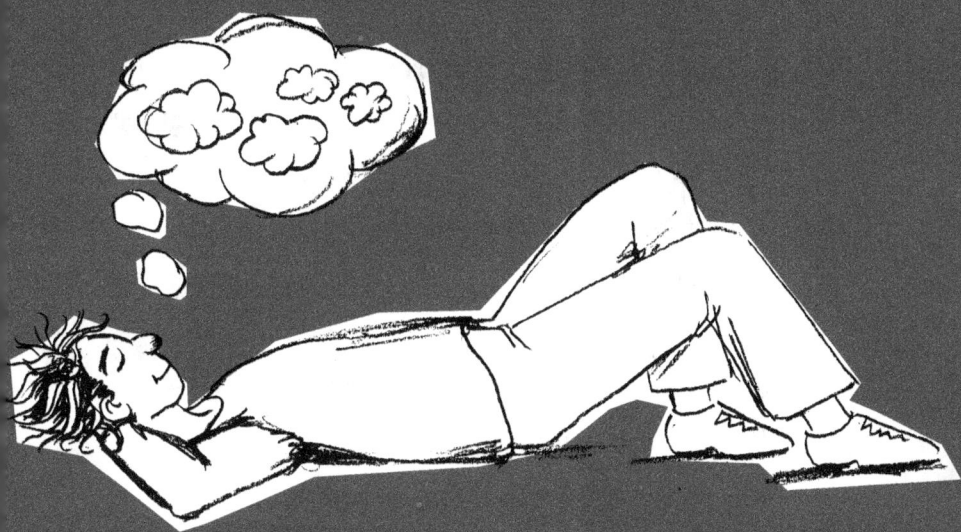

This exercise is thought as a supplementary but not nec-essary add-on application. You might add it to the previous mental formulas, when you are very familiar with them.

With this supplementary exercise, you reveal another dimension of yourself. As usual, begin by conducting the previous exercises. It is now easy to concentrate and to get connected to the inner resources all by itself.

When you know all the previous exercises by heart after 4 to 6 weeks, you can select one of the following "free" phrases if it feels real to you. (But only one and then for some weeks the same; otherwise the training will be too long or too "changy".)

I love and accept myself (and my body) the way I am.
I am guided by the divine.
I am happy that everything is the way it is.
I am a happy, grateful person.

If you want to, you can replace or complement these sentences using your own images that are suited to your personal situation. But it is very important that the content remains consistent with your reality.

If other thoughts arise, allow them to flow freely (if unpleasant thoughts or feelings come, just let them drift away, like clouds in the sky) and concentrate only on your phrases.

Feel like a child – simple, naïve and loving!

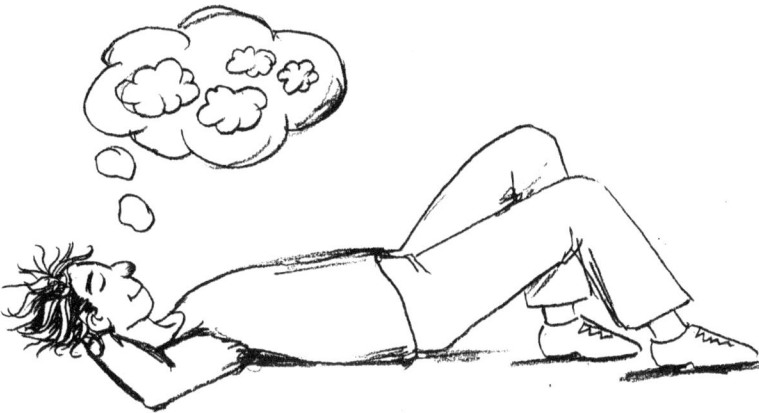

Congratulations

On the previous pages you have gotten to know a method of training that gives you access to the deciding mechanisms of your subconscious. You now know the language to use to communicate with this inexhaustible source of strength, with this powerful helper inside you, and how to take advantage of it – and that is through the connection between images and intense feelings.

For us brain-oriented people, learning this language is not always easy. It is like learning a foreign language. The more you practice, the better it works, the larger your "vocabulary" becomes and the less misunderstandings there are. This also applies to learning *TrophoTraining*®: in spite of its simplicity, "practice makes perfect!"

The best strategy to integrate *TrophoTraining*® in your life is to include it into your daily routine, like brushing your teeth. You can look forward to the exciting discoveries that you will continue to make! Every day you will see that you feel better and better, more peaceful and more serene, and that you are a happier, more self-confident person. Along with the exercises, also read these theoretical explanations from time to time.

Experience has shown that most people only realize the enormous significance of the principles that *TrophoTraining*® is founded on bit by bit. Knowing them, however, is very important for lasting training success and can be expanded through the right courses. Be patient, take all the time you need and please do not forget: "No sweet without sweat!"

Because *TrophoTraining®* is based on Dr. Udo Derbolowsky's psychopädie®, I have provided a short overview of the key possibilities and practical applications of the psychopaedic approach in the appendix. If you

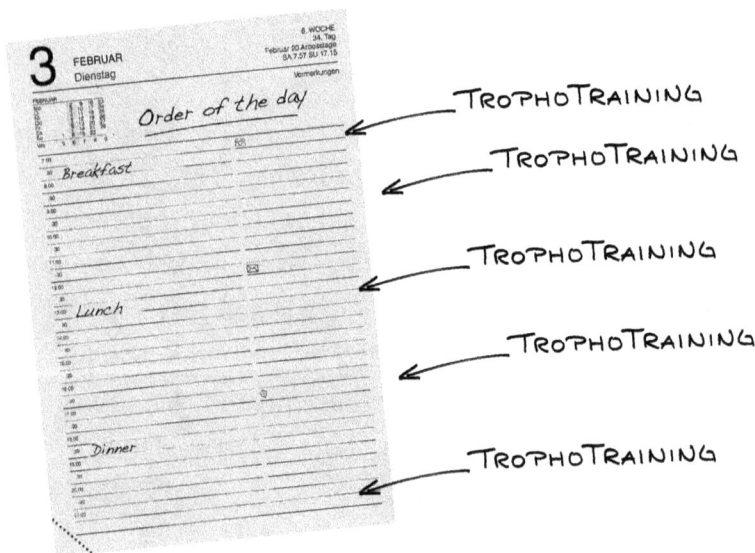

would like to know more about the subject or have questions, write us a short message and you will receive the
requested information.

TrophoTraining® Institute • Im Tann 16 • D-82110 Germering
Phone: 0049-89-84-75-71 • Fax: 0049-89-8-94-81-21
www.trophotraining.de • info@trophotraining.de

Appendix

Dr. Udo Derbolowsky's Psychopädie®

The term **psychopädie** is composed of the words psycho- (Greek: psyche = soul) and -paedia (Greek: paideia = education, learning). First and foremost, psychopädie deals with the connections and possibilities of life, work, partnership, and communication problems. Psychopädie nurtures behavior and nobleness of heart, from which you can immediately introduce the results into your life and how you deal with yourself and others.

Psychopädie teaches you how to lovingly interact with yourself, the people around you, God, and the world. It shows how giving and taking can be held in joyful balance. Psychopädie is a balanced synthesis of the most important discoveries in psychology, psychotherapy and psychoanalysis. At the same time, it also uses traditional wisdom from the greatest philosophers of humankind and is deeply rooted in the belief of a loving creator. As a pragmatic, scientifically founded path to discovery, it serves to free and develop one's own personal potential and the operationalized implementation of the biblical commandment of love in everyday life. It allows personal potential to unfold and grow stronger.

Psychopädie was developed by the doctor, psychotherapist, and well-known psychoanalyst, Dr. Udo Derbolowsky,
based on over 50 years of his practical experience and
research. Both its content and structure are free from the
influence of any secular or religious organizations.

Psychopädie is also distinguished by the fact that it offers a reliable and easily applicable method to recognize the patterns and conditioning within oneself and produces the desired changes. Work-related examples of application are:

- Additional qualifications, i.e. for doctors, health practitioners, teachers, ministers and pastors, educators and counselors, trainers, etc.
- Counseling, teaching and supervisory work (also as self-employed psychopaedists)
- Healthcare and rehabilitation work
- Leadership and management activities
- Sports and recreation (inclusion of mental potential)

Private Akademie für Psychopädie Dr. Derbolowsky
Im Tann 16 · D-82110 Germering
Phone 0049-89-84-75-71 · Fax 0049-89-8-94-81-21
www.trophotraining.de · info@trophotraining.de

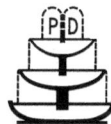

Recommended reading

(see also www.psychopaedica.de)

- Udo and Jakob Derbolowsky: Liebenswert bist Du immer - so schützen Sie Ihre seelische Gesundheit; Junfermann, Paderborn, 3. Aufl. 2007, ISBN 978-3-387387-473-2
- Udo and Regina Derbolowsky: Atem ist Leben, Psychopädica, Germering (Bod) 2. Aufl. 2005, ISBN 978-3-933400-10-9
- Udo Derbolowsky: Kränkung, Krankheit, Heilung, Neuromedizin, Hersfeld, 5. Aufl. 2006, ISBN 978-3-930-926-06-0
- Jakob Derbolowsky: TrophoTraining® - So fühle ich mich wohl, Hörbuch-CD, Psychopädica, Germering, 3. Unveränderte Aufl. 2008, ISBN 978-3-933400-06-2
- Jakob Derbolowsky/Ilse Middendorf: Psycho-somatische Störungen, Psychopädica, Germering, 2. Aufl. (Bod), 1999, ISBN 978-3-933400-04-8

About the author

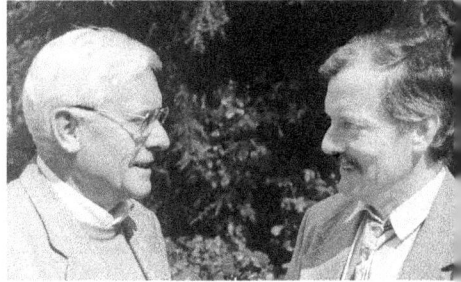

Dr. Jakob Derbolowsky runs the Private Academy for Psycho-paedia and the Tropho-Training-Institute. He has been working as a doctor and psychotherapist for 35 years. For the past 30 years, he has been training and counseling people working in healthcare and education as well as business and management on psychopaedic themes.

Dr. Jakob Derbolowsky with his father Dr. Udo Derbolowsky, the founder of Psychopadie

Several thousand people have participated in his courses and seminars over the years, not to mention those who have listened to his lectures and regular radio show "Alltagswerkstatt in der Lebenshilfe" on the radio station Horeb (www.horeb.org). He has participated in health shows on different television stations (ZDF, mdr, BR), in the German newspapers' medical tour, and worked with various magazines. He is well known outside of his field through his scientific work and as an author and publisher of books.

"Transcend the shell and discover the
pearl that you really are."

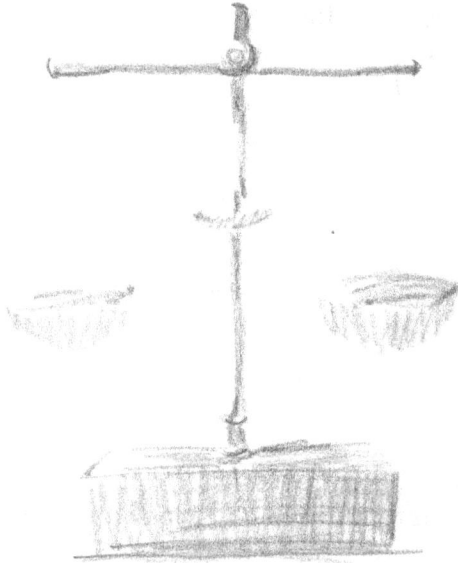

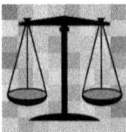

TrophoTraining® Institute • Im Tann 16 • D-82110 Germering
www.trophotraining.de • info@trophotraining.de

www.ingramcontent.com/pod-product-compliance
Lightning Source LLC
Chambersburg PA
CBHW070931270326
41927CB00011B/2816